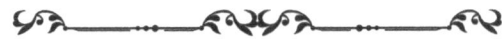

A LONG ROAD
TO THE RIGHT KIND
OF CARE

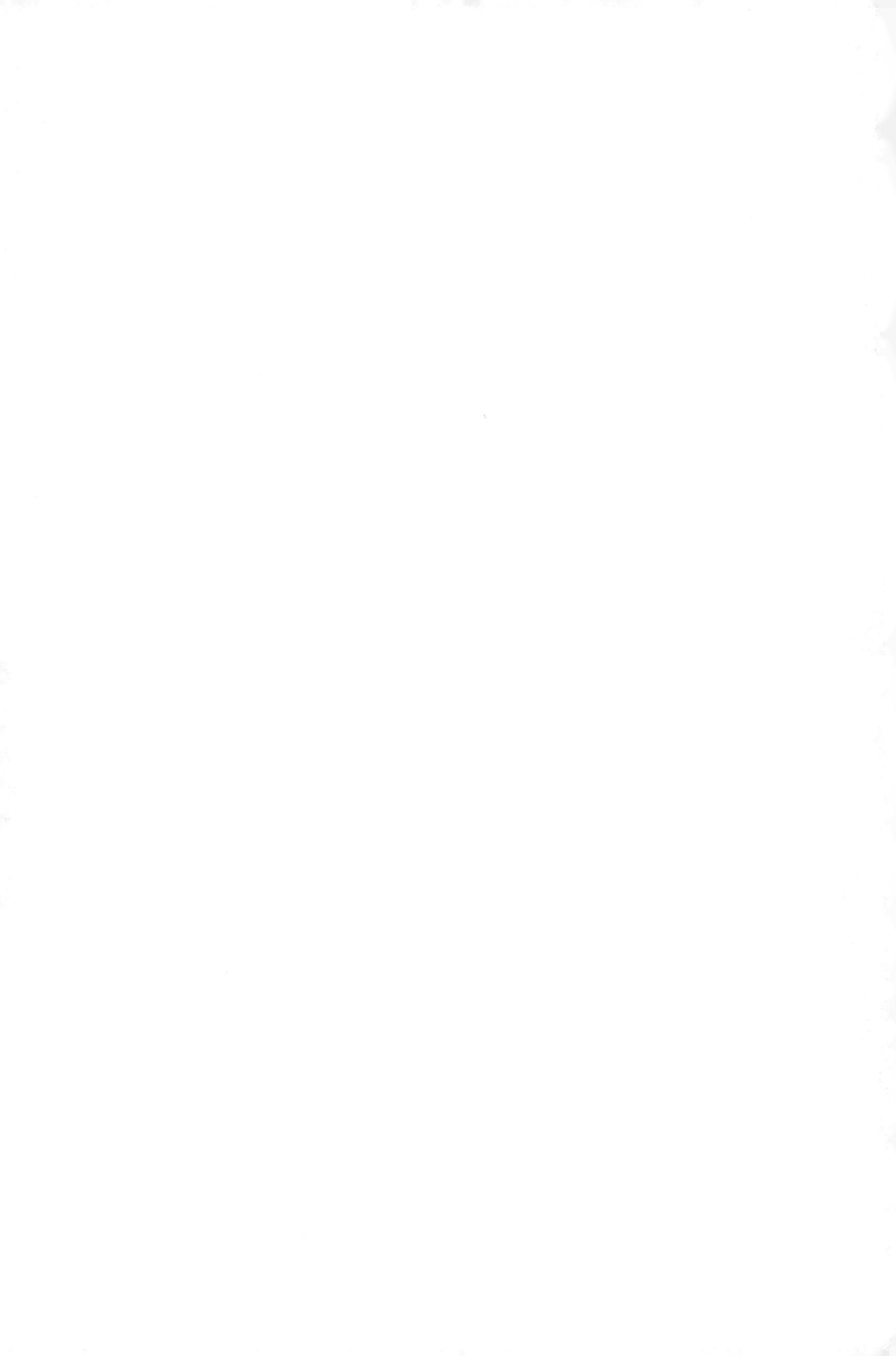

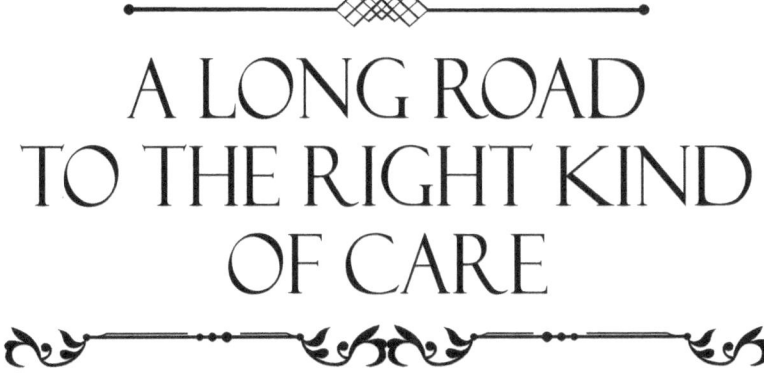

A LONG ROAD
TO THE RIGHT KIND
OF CARE

ALEXANDER ROGERSON, MD

Library of Congress Control Number: 2017903048
ISBN: Hardcover   978-1-5245-8764-2
               Softcover   978-1-5245-8763-5
               eBook   978-1-5245-8814-4

Rev. date: 02/27/2017

To order additional copies of this book, contact:
Xlibris
1-888-795-4274
www.Xlibris.com
Orders@Xlibris.com
756012

My long experience in the practice of medicine is, I think, unusual, and I feel I should speak out.

I was born ninety-four years ago at home and delivered by a physician, although many, at that time, were delivered by midwives, and many of the mothers succumbed to "childbed fever," and the babies, fairly often, did not survive. Almost all babies were breastfed by their mothers, or a few were fed by "wet nurses" if the family was wealthy and the mother could not feed the baby.

My education was in private and not public schools, and was unisexual after the sixth grade. I, however, was a so-called day student and lived at home, whereas a large majority of the students were boarding students and lived in dormitories at the school. After the usual twelve grades of education, I attended college at Harvard, already equipped with the desire to become a doctor. I had great admiration for our family doctor, and I was impressed with the respect that my family and many others had for him.

Because of the war, my college attendance was only two-and-a-half years, and since I had completed all the academic requirements, I was accepted early to Harvard Medical School. The army, then, drafted me before I received my college degree, with the agreement that I would be sent to medical school when my class opened, I was sent to Camp Grant in Rockford, Illinois, for basic training. This was a medical department camp and was filled with about seventy-five thousand soldiers. Most of the men and officers belonged to religious groups that did not believe in warfare but were willing to serve as medics. The captain of our company was a Seventh-Day Adventist, and there were quite a few in our camp. I was assigned to a tent, which held six of us.

This was my first exposure to many folk who had not been raised as I had been, and to an environment that was, to me, most unusual. There were a small group of us who were "premeds" waiting for our classes to begin. Our corporal greeted us by referring to us in an unusual manner. "All right, you fuckups, start picking up all them butts." And so we began to pick up all the cigarette butts scattered around the grounds.

Our cots were very simple with straw mattresses. We were issued very simple uniforms and equipment, and were assigned to a basic training company. My tent mates included a man with a wooden leg and a guy who had made his living as a hypnotist in civilian life. I wondered about the wooden leg and found the hypnotist fascinating. Some of the officers in our company wanted to see him perform, but the captain, a Seventh-Day Adventist, forbid him to do so, as his religious beliefs were that hypnotism was the work of the devil and that was it. Our tent companion gave a few secret demonstrations anyway.

Basic training was somewhat dull but was enlivened by various incidents and classes. We were taught how to retrieve the wounded under fire by running with stretchers and falling to the ground on command and how to use bandages to stop bleeding and to carry the wounded to battalion aid stations. Our tent mate with the wooden leg couldn't run well with the stretcher and was quite clumsy. The sergeant picked this up and asked what the problem was. When he said that he had a wooden leg, the sergeant said, "Don't give me that bull," and we all said "No, Sarge, he does and puts under the bed at night."

The sergeant said, "How the hell did you ever get drafted?" It seems that no one at the induction center had asked him, and he was not examined below the waist.

This was not an uncommon occurrence. The draft boards had a quota, and they often filled it with handicapped draftees. The expectation was that the army would not accept them, but they were never examined again unless they went on sick call.

I didn't realize that if a company came by with an unfurled flag, I was to stop what I was doing and salute while they passed. I thus didn't, and the company was restricted for a week with no leave. I was unpopular, for a bit, with my comrades but managed to survive. Kitchen police (KP) and latrine duty were the usual punishments for various kinds of behavior, and one of our premeds, while on latrine duty, rigged the toilets with string so he could lift all the lids at once. On inspection, when called to attention, he lifted all the lids. He got quite used to latrine and KP duty.

One of our premeds named Dunkle was a nice guy but a "nerd"; he used fancy words and was a bit chubby. We did a lot of marching, and the corporals made him be road guard so he had to run out at each crossing, and they also teased him a lot. He did no complaining and carried on as best he could.

One day word came down from headquarters that he was to report, because his father, General Dunkle, wished to see him. There was consternation in the ranks. He reported, came back, and never said a word. The rest of us, of course, said, "Why didn't you tell us your old man was a major general?" But he just smiled. Needless to say, all teasing, etc., ceased.

We also had a drill team, of which I was a member, which performed at events such as halftime at football games. If they were close, we were marched out; otherwise we were driven by truck. On one occasion, I became ill on the way back from a football game. It wasn't bad, but I was hospitalized for a few days, and was assigned for a day to paint a hospital room along with another patient. An officer came by and complained that we were doing a lousy job as painters. We both told him we were not painters, and explained that we were in basic training, in the hospital, as patients, and about to return to our units. He went off mumbling about the crazy army.

After basic training, I was assigned to guarding German and Italian prisoners of war. About fifty thousand Germans and four thousand Italians were sent to our camp after the battle, in the Middle East, in "El Alamein." It seems that the British fleet had blockaded the German ships that supplied General Rommel's Africa Corp and the Italian Arrete Corp, and so they had almost no fuel or ammunition for the tanks. When General Montgomery sent out the scotish bagpipers (referred to as the ladies from hell), the night before the battle, they knew that the next day he would attack, and so they all surrendered when he did so the next morning. It is said that Prime Minister Churchill asked President Roosevelt what he was going to do with two hundred and fifty thousand prisoners of war. Roosevelt suggested that he send them to us.

Most Americans don't realize that we had two hundred and fifty thousand of them scattered over the United States. We had to open the trunks of cars visiting Camp Grant because some of the Italian prisoners were found being smuggled out by the American ladies.

Many of the prisoners spoke English, and so we exchanged a lot of information. Some had been in the rescue group that tried to break through the Russian Army to rescue the German troops in the Siege of Stalingrad. Others had been with the German troops in the Alps and ran into Japanese American troops of the 442, a regiment that was entirely of Japanese extraction. It was the most highly decorated regiment in the army and received twenty-some medals of honor. Their motto was "Go for broke."

The Germans, as prisoners of war, told me they asked, "Who are you and why are you here?" They were laughingly told that Japan had declared war on Germany. Since their families had been sent to camps in California, even though they were American citizens, it seemed weird that these young men would be in the army.

It's not necessary to be an American citizen to be an enlisted man in our army, however. One of my classmates at college was distantly connected to the Japanese royal family. The FBI hunted him down and found that he had been drafted, and was at Fort Devons in Massachusetts. It was suggested that he could work as an interpreter.

He, however, pointed out that he was third-generation American and didn't speak Japanese.

The German and Italian prisoners did not know much about us at all. They thought that they were sent to our camp in a closed train so they wouldn't see the bombing. We told them we had not been bombed. They had no idea how large a country we were in area and population, that we were fighting two wars, and that we had millions of people in the armed forces. Our camp, with about seventy-five thousand medical department soldiers, seemed huge to them, as did our obvious industrial power.

After guarding prisoners, I was sent back to Fort Devons and worked as an orderly on the violently insane ward in the hospital until my medical school class opened. I found it difficult to understand how these men had found their way into the army to begin with, but there they were.

I arrived at medical school, in World War II, as a "private first class U.S. army" (a promotion). (The navy students were midshipmen).

Medical school, in the first two years, was entirely academic, with the exception of human anatomy, which involved the dissection of a corpse by a team of four of us first-year students. I was one of four in my class to be selected as a "prosector," and we had to dissect another corpse for the use of the professor of anatomy in his lectures. The first two years of medical school were referred to "as a gauntlet to be run to prove that you had the ability to become a physician." The courses were academic and included subjects such as physiology (how a normal human body works), pharmacology (drugs), bacteriology (how bacteria grow and infect humans), pathology (abnormal physiology produced by disease), and parasitology (other biological beings that attack humans).

It was quite obvious during those first two years that our knowledge of human illness, although much better than that of previous generations, was not sufficient to alter the course of most diseases to any great extent. We did have ether as an anesthetic for surgery, and sulfanilamide was the only antibiotic available and was not very effective. A few drugs were truly effective, such as insulin (for diabetes) and digitalis (for heart failure). We also had basic knowledge of bacteria and evidence that they caused many infectious diseases. This allowed us to introduce "asepsis" (hand washing and sterilization of instruments, gowns, rubber gloves, and any equipment used in the operating room) and antisepsis (using chemicals to sterilize the environment especially in operating rooms). Antisepsis was introduced by Dr. Lister, who had developed the idea of chemical antisepsis. The chemicals used in the operating rooms were often harmful, particularly to those administering the ether for anesthesia, and not very effective, and so they were no longer used by the time I started my medical education. A few antiseptics, however, such as alcohol, mercurochrome, and tincture of iodine were used on the skin. Viruses were not known as such, but we had the beginnings of immunization for viral illnesses such as rabies and the use of the vaccinia virus (cow pox) as a vaccine to prevent smallpox. In 1945, penicillin came into some general use. It had just been developed and would soon be produced in large amounts for more general use. It was an extremely effective antibiotic against certain bacteria and led to the end of specialists in the treatment of syphilis.

Polio illuminates our current medical problems and their hope for solution. It seemed, originally, to be a disease of advanced countries and not of third world countries, where it was called "infantile paralysis." It was rare in underdeveloped countries and seemed to occur mostly in infants. One of the first large outbreaks was in Sweden, among adults, as well as infants and children. In industrial societies, adults were more likely to develop severe disease and worse paralysis. As time went by, we learned a lot. First, we discovered that it is a contagious disease spread by intestinal carriers, and is caused by a virus, which was first grown on animal tissue by Dr. Enders at Harvard University. This allowed the development of a vaccine to prevent the disease. Secondly, we found that antiviral medications are not an answer to most viral infections. Viruses grow inside cells, unlike most bacteria, however, and vaccines to prevent a viral illness are the main answer to viral illnesses. Immunizations, on a worldwide basis, are the main protection against such infections, and may lead to their elimination, as smallpox has been eradicated, and measles, mumps, rubella, and polio have been greatly reduced. Thirdly, only when people are deathly afraid of a disease will they pursue immunizations, and we now have a large group of people who are more afraid of immunizations than the various diseases, and dangerous anti-scientific beliefs are spread by the Internet. MMR vaccine is wrongly believed to cause autism, polio vaccine to cause sterility, etc. Thus problems that we thought we had solved long ago are not. Also an interesting problem of our modern society is the way Mother Nature works. In third world countries, almost all babies catch polio within the first few months of life, but because they have antibodies from their mother transmitted by the placenta and breastmilk, it is unusual to see poliomyelitis as a disease in these populations. In developed countries, protection from the immunized mother is less likely, and, of course, not at all from the un-immunized. Also, as mentioned above, the older you are, the more likely you are to develop a more severe disease with permanent paralysis. The developing countries such as India, Pakistan, and most African countries thus depend on the polio vaccine to eliminate the disease from their countries. The Sabin live polio vaccine is used because it spreads from person to person. In the USA, we have reverted to the dead Salk vaccine, and thus, those who have compromised immune systems will not, even though it is very rare, get polio from the vaccine. However, people immunized with the dead vaccine may still can carry the live virus in their intestines. Many people who refuse immunizations think they are protected by the surrounding immunized populations, but this is not true for quite a few diseases that are only an airline ride away.

Vitamins as necessary ingredients of foods had been known, but not identified, for many years. They were named in 1912 by a man named Funk. In the 1920s, vitamins A, E, C, and K were identified as essential to the human diet. By the 1940s, we were well aware that all these substances were essential to prevent and treat many illnesses and abnormal conditions.

For pediatricians, baby formulas were of great interest. The industrial revolution wiped out the availability of wet nurses, and substitutes for breastmilk were attempted. No one had any idea of how complicated the composition of breastmilk really was. Starting in the 1800s, various combinations of cow's milk, water, cream, and sugar or honey were concocted, which led to lots of problems, such as scurvy and rickets, for example, from vitamin deficiencies, and infections, such as tuberculosis, from raw milk. Malnutrition and the wrong ratios of ingredients led to the death of many babies. In 1845 the rubber nipple was developed, and in 1867, Von Leibig developed what he called soluble food for infants. None of this worked too well, and it was shown, in 1922, that of bottle babies, one in five lived through the first year, and of breastfed, twenty-nine out of thirty. Many used honey in the formula, and a significant number of babies developed botulism from the honey. Ironic that we now use the toxin, Botox, cosmetically. In the 1930s, pasteurized milk, evaporated milk, and the icebox revolutionized things. When I started in pediatrics in the late 1940s, we all used evaporated milk in almost all the formulas. It was so convenient and it worked well. "No teat to pull, no dung to fling, just punch two holes in the 'gol darn' thing." The formula was one can of evaporated milk (13 ounces), 17 ounces of water, and 3 tablespoons of Karo syrup. By the 1950s most people were using premixed formulas such as Simulac or Enfamil. They also were switching to disposable diapers.

In the last two years of medical school, in addition to more academic scientific courses, we were exposed to much that was not academic, and it changed my attitudes and opinions in many ways. (Actually, we did four years in three because we were in the army in wartime and had no summer vacations.)

In our third year, we began to be exposed to the actual medical care of patients. I soon reached the conclusion that my original ideas of becoming a surgeon were not appropriate for my abilities. The dean at Harvard fortified this position and felt that I was much more suited to academic medicine, research, or medical practice. One day, I watched an attending physician, while making rounds, change the course of treatment in an unusual manner. He called the resident, in charge of a newly admitted patient in heart failure, over to talk to him. The resident team was very busy doing the few therapeutic treatments available at that time, most of which did little more than to make the lady very uncomfortable and prolong her existence. He said to him, "Doctor, have you found a way to leave this world other than feet first? Let's make her comfortable."

The idea of "hospice" had not been even been considered at that time.

As medical students, we were given some well-supervised duties usually on the wards in the public hospitals. One of our classes involved surgery, with ether anesthesia, on dogs as patients; another was giving ether as an anesthetic during the delivery of a baby, or as leg holders during a delivery. Previous classes of students had been required to deliver a baby at home in order to complete their obstetrical rotation. Because of the war, and our early acceptance to medical school, a few of us were quite young. One of my classmates was still under twenty-one in his fourth year, and an exception had to be made for him, because Massachusetts law required one to be over twenty-one to deliver a baby. We were no longer, as the previous classes had been, required to deliver a baby at home. Those who had done home deliveries had all sorts of tales to tell about such deliveries and the problems involved. One delivery involved a baby that was stillborn, and thus, the necessity of the student to carry the body in a bag back to the city hospital on the Boston subway. The home deliveries were carried out only on the many multiparous ladies who were delivering at home. The delivery by students required little skill and was considered quite acceptable.

By spending time on the various hospital services, we learned about the many specialties of medical care, and this gave us an idea about what we might like to do in the medical field. Our rotations to the various services in the teaching hospitals also exposed us to a variety of patients from all over the different sections of Boston.

During our medical school years, almost all of us were in the army or the navy. We graduated in 1947, and the war ended in 1945, but we were not discharged until well into our fourth year. Some of us were sent to school directly from the army, and since we had been drafted in the middle of college and had been in the army for many months, we were knowledgeable. Others were placed in the army or navy on entering school. The navy students were midshipmen, as at Annapolis, but we were not cadets, as at West Point; we were promoted to private first class and were part of the Army Specialized Training Corps (ASTP). As such, we wore an insignia, which we referred to as the "flaming chamber pot," and were berated by the chant, "Take down your service flag, mother, your son's in the ASTP."

We also had to rise at seven every morning and assemble to "sound off" and be counted. We designated one of us to answer roll call for all of us. Our commanding officer was a major who came from the Chicago's West Side, and he was great and not very strict. However, the colonel at Harvard College heard about us and demanded an inspection. He gave a number of orders about various things he wanted done, including textbooks arranged in order of size, nothing hung from windows, reville each morning, and beds made up after revile, etc. Major Rosenguard is reported to have said, "Colonel, what you're ordering will not work. We are not training these men to be soldiers; we are training them to be doctors, and you come from West Point and I come from the Chicago West Side." At any rate we had no more trouble.

The incoming class in our fourth year contained women for the first time at Harvard Medical School, and so the medical world changed. I graduated in 1947 and decided to become a pediatrician. I was accepted at Boston Children's Hospital as a first-year resident. To be a board-certified pediatrician required three years of training at a teaching hospital. The third-year residents supervised a team of four or five first-year residents run by a second-year resident. The first-year residents admitted patients and performed the work involved in making a diagnosis of the child's illness and starting treatment needed to help Mother Nature cure the patient. This involved a medical history, physical exam, doing the various laboratory tests, X-rays, and requesting consultations with specialists if indicated.

General pediatric practitioners in the community donated a month of their time to act as "attending physicians." This meant that they made daily rounds with the team and made basic decisions about the care of patients who were admitted, without a physician, to oversee their care in the hospital. Most patients had their own doctor who oversaw such care and gave orders as to what should be done. These attending physicians were not paid and were those who enjoyed teaching young residents about general pediatric practice and were experienced in the treatment of the various diseases and problems. It also helped to keep the attendings up to date in the care of serious problems seen all the time in teaching hospitals and rarely in general practice. The residents, at that time, were given room, board, and food, but they also were not paid. The state of medical care then was such that, although we had little in the way of drugs that could alter the course of an illness, we could help to maintain the normal physiology of the body and allow a disease to run its course without death or great damage.

Penicillin appeared during my resident training and made a huge difference in the treatment of many patients. It also changed the illnesses admitted to the hospital, since many were now treated as outpatients. An example of this was rheumatic fever, a serious illness that was an immune system reaction to streptococcal infections. We had a whole hospital devoted to this disease. If streptococcal infections were treated early on with penicillin, it did not develop. So successful was this that, when in later years we admitted a patient with symptoms of this disease to the hospital, I was the only one who had ever seen a patient with such symptoms. Tuberculosis, found even in Egyptian mummies as far back as 2800 BC, was almost always lethal. The bacterium was discovered by Robert Koch in 1822, but no treatment was available except for palliative care.

Another hospital in our community had a whole ward devoted to the treatment of Scottish war brides who developed the disease from using raw milk. The milk in Scotland was not pasteurized, and bovine TB was thus common in the cattle in Scotland. In 1940 a drug, actinomycin, was discovered to kill TB bacteria but was too toxic to use. In 1949, isoniazid was found to be very effective, and the tuberculosis sanitariums began to fade away. Antibiotics seemed to be miracles in our care of the sick, but the evolution of resistant bacteria has changed the picture. An unusual problem developed in our female children being treated for tuberculosis. They were developing signs of early puberty at a much too early age. It was discovered that the drug companies manufacturing isoniazid were also processing a powerful female drug hormone (stilbestrol) on the same machines, and the machines were not being properly cleaned after each drug was processed.

Our greatest improvement in medical care was, however, in prevention. Immunizations against serious and often fatal diseases had eliminated some of our scourges such as diphtheria, tetanus, smallpox, and whooping cough. As might be expected, families were very frightened by hospitals and often did not seek care early in the course of illness. After all, hospitals were places where people died. "Good doctors" were those that could provide comfort and information to parents, and hope and reassurance when needed. Also we could control pain and avoid unnecessary treatments that were not called for. During my final year as a resident, cortisone, in the form of ACTH, a hormone, which stimulates the adrenal gland to produce more cortisone, also appeared as an available treatment and this then began to change the course of many illnesses. These were inflammatory diseases, due to the reaction of our immune system to inflame human cells. They were numerous, and we really did not understand them or what caused them. Thus we had almost no idea how to treat them beyond the use of aspirin, which seemed to help somewhat.

After three years of training in three different hospitals and six months of being a fourth-year or "chief resident" at Philadelphia Children's Hospital, I was again drafted by the army due to the shortage of army doctors during the Korean War. This time I was an officer (first lieutenant), the lowest rank for a doctor in the army. I was sent to Fort

Ord in California, where I ran a large pediatric clinic. I was there for two and a half years, and I learned a great deal about army medicine as a doctor rather than as a medical department soldier. Specialists in internal medicine are out of their field, to some extent, in the army. The commandant of the Fort Ord Hospital told me when he discovered that I was a pediatrician, "You'll find that these men are just children grown big." That is, of course, the truth. They suffer, mostly, from pediatric problems, infectious diseases, and traumatic injuries, not the degenerative diseases of the geriatric population.

I was placed in charge of the pediatric clinic because I was board qualified, and my companion, although a captain, was not. The army generally functions on rank, however, and this can lead to problems. An example of this was our surgeon who was a lieutenant colonel. A young child was admitted with what I thought was a ruptured appendix. The colonel did not agree with my diagnosis and tried to get my captain colleague to agree with him.

The full colonel, who was the head of the internal medical department and who had confidence in my abilities, told him, "If Rogerson says operate, you operate." He did, the child did have a ruptured appendix, and all went well. It seems that the lieutenant colonel had had other difficulties, which the army solved in its usual manner; they transferred him and made him a club officer in Korea. The army, at that time, assumed that all doctors were equal, and thus they were often placed in situations for which they were not trained. Good heads of departments overrode such circumstances when they could. During the Korean War, the army was very short of doctors, and thus attempts were made to shut down the pediatric clinic and transferus to the medical service. The general in command of Fort Ord would not allow this, however. A few times, my colleague and I would be transferred in the morning and by noon, be back in the pediatric clinic. The general is reported to have said, "We promised to take care of the children and wives of the soldiers overseas, and I want the pediatric clinic open." All of us were required to take sick call, and a friend of mine, a psychiatrist, was seeing a young soldier who seemed quite sick and asked me to look at him. I did and suggested that the young man needed first to take off his clothes. He was indeed sick and had the typical rash of a bloodstream infection with the meningitis bacteria. We, of course, sent him off to the hospital, but there was little to be done, and he died the next day.

Meningitis is a problem with large groups that come from all over and are held in barracks or dormitories. There is now a vaccine for the most common meningitis bacteria, and is suggested for use on army recruits and college freshmen.

The army had a number of men in medical schools, and on graduation they were given the rank of first lieutenant and sent for a one-year internship. After the internship, they were promoted to captain and sent to Korea as physicians, usually in battalion aid stations. After a year or so, they were often promoted to major and sent to posts in the United

States. Since they had little training in regular medical care, it was hard to assign them. At any rate, I got two of them in pediatric clinic for a month or two. A major general came down from San Francisco for an inspection and asked to see the pediatric clinic. I was busy doing a procedure on a small baby, and so he looked and talked a bit and when I was finished, he called me over and asked if I was in charge of the clinic. I told him that I was, and he asked my rank.

"How is it that you are the head and in command when there are two majors and a captain working here?"

I explained that I was the only one who was board qualified in pediatrics and thus had been placed in charge. He smiled and said, "You know, Doctor, the army is crazy."

A humorous incident occurred when the full colonel in charge of the hospital was arguing with a new draftee about hemophilia. This is a blood clotting failure, which occurs only in men and is a genetic defect carried on the sex, or X chromosome, by women. The colonel was of the opinion that women could not have the disease. From the practical point of view, this was correct, but the new doctor pointed out that it was not always true. The colonel was going to verify his point by looking it up in Cecil's medical textbook The doctor replied, "That won't help, Colonel, because I wrote the article on hemophilia in Cecil."

The doctor's draft brought in quite a few interesting academic physicians.

The war ended and I accepted a place with the Berkeley Pediatric Group and a half-time appointment with the University of California in San Francisco as an instructor. The pediatric group was unusual, as the head of the group had decided, in 1993, along with his wife, also a pediatrician, to limit the practice to patients who paid by the year. The medical association, needless to say, didn't like this, and he was labeled a communist. The people in Berkeley did like it, and when I joined the group, there were four physicians and an additional office in the nearby town of Lafayette. Dr. Jennings, the head of the group, was about fifty years ahead of his time. One of the members,

Dr. Bruyn, was a full-time faculty member at UCSF and the group had a high ranking in the quality of its care. Although we were not charging enough to make as much money as those in pay-per-visit practice, we were very attractive to the families in town and were doing well. We had our own laboratory, which allowed us to do blood counts and bacteriology, and we used the hospital facilities for X-rays and blood chemistries, which we did not cover. If a child had to be hospitalized, our visits to the hospital were covered. Our visits to the hospitals for newborns were also covered, and also my exchange transfusions for newborns, although they were rare. We also developed a program for the home care of newborn babies who developed jaundice and required light therapy. This home therapy, practiced over a period of many years, worked very well for our group. The photo therapy was required for only two or three days, but the standard practice was to readmit the newborn to the hospital for the light treatment. This made nursing difficult and an inconvenient separation of mother and baby. The program started because a father, in the practice, asked why they couldn't do this at home. I couldn't think of a reason why not, and so we set up the light machine in the home and arranged visits by our nurses. After thirteen years, we published a paper in one of the pediatric journals. Although it was well received, it did not convince many pediatricians to try it. The admission to the hospital was too convenient for the physicians, and like house calls, this kind of home care was not financially productive.

Medical care in the United States is focused on the treatment of illness and is increasingly hospital based. A general practice in the outside community, especially pediatric general care, is primarily involved with preventive and developmental medicine. Our patients usually leave us when they go off to college or start a separate life.

Pay per visit, for-profit medical care, is not really suited to healthcare for the young, and copayments and deductibles can put a terrible burden on medical care for any age. Although we were not looked upon kindly by the medical association, the arrival of Kaiser medical care refocused their attention. I also noted, as my practice grew, that I was concerned primarily with well-child care. "An ounce of prevention really is worth a pound of cure." Examinations of healthy babies and children and conversations about development and preventive care had little to do with illness. Therefore, most of my time was spent on subjects that had not much to do with what I had learned in medical school or my hospital training. The better our preventive care, the fewer seriously ill patients we saw, and when we did, we saw them early in the course of their illness. Relatively few of our patients required hospitalization, and thus, I was treating minor illnesses and practicing mostly preventive medicine.

After two years, I gave up my instructor status at UCSF and devoted myself to my practice. I did remain on the clinical faculty, without pay, and taught residents at Oakland Children's Hospital for a month each year. I also served on various hospital committees.

When I started teaching, in 1953, our residents were almost all male, and our attending physicians were all practitioners in the community. As time went by, the number of women residents increased and the general pediatric practitioners who volunteered to be attending physicians decreased until all, except me, were gone. When I left, after fifty-four years of attending, the residents were mostly women, about 80 percent. Their approach to medical care was different from the standard male approach, and they faced extra problems in adjusting their lives to medical practice, family raising, and their roles in the community. Meanwhile, the hospital became increasingly separated from clinical medical care on the outside. Fifty to sixty years ago, if a patient was admitted to the hospital, his or her community physician wrote the orders for care, told the residents what he or she wanted done, and was responsible for the care while in the hospital. When I stopped my "teaching rounds" at Children's Hospital, the general pediatric practitioners were gone and a new specialty had arisen. The new specialists were called hospitalists, and if a child was sent to the hospital, his or her doctor no longer cared for her or him while in the hospital. A hospitalist took over the care. In addition the residents thus lost almost all contact with outside practitioners. The residents, who are now unionized and paid, generally decide to become hospitalists, sub specialists, or emergency room physicians. For women, especially, these are attractive choices, because one's time can be scheduled, and this allows them to handle their multiple responsibilities. When I started practice, I had the responsibility of earning enough to raise five children. My wife had a full-time job managing a household and the children, and I could not have done without her. The hospitals also decided to make a few residents attending physicians, to replace the attending physicians from the community. In the past, one resident was chosen from the third-year residents to be the fourth-year or chief resident and supervise the resident teams, as I had been at Philadelphia Children's Hospital, but not to be the attending physician. The attending physicians are now fourth-year residents or hospitalists. If a resident wanted to find out what community general practice was like, she or he needed to spend time in an office or clinic.

We had a few residents who spent a month of their rotation in our office for that reason. One of the residents from Oakland Children's Hospital came to our office for a month to see what private practice was like. We were talking at lunchtime, and she happened to comment that her father had been a prisoner of war in World War II. It turned out that he was in the "Wermacht" and was in Benicia, California. He got bored and decided to leave and see the country. He had no green card, and he picked up jobs as he traveled along. Eventually he returned to the camp in Benicia and found that they had no record of him! He eventually was repatriated but returned as an immigrant and became a cardiologist in Los Angeles, and this was his daughter. I often wondered how many of the German prisoners of war had come back as immigrants.

Teaching hospitals thus have little contact with the outside community, except in their emergency rooms and clinics, and the patients seen in their clinics and admitted to the hospital are very different from those seen in a practice. As a general pediatric practitioner, what I might see once every two to three years might be seen every two to three weeks in a teaching hospital. For example, Dr. Farber, at Boston Children's Hospital, was so involved with the treatment of pediatric cancer that he had a whole ward of patients that were not expected to survive. The resident teams, in training, also handle their patients in the hospital differently now. Instead of "making rounds," as the attending physicians used to do with the residents every day, each first-year resident checks his patients in the morning prior to a meeting of the resident team. At the meeting, held in a special room, the second-year resident is in charge, and the third-year resident sits with the computer. Each patient is discussed and the third-year resident looks up the laboratory and X-ray reports, notes from specialists who have been asked to see the patient, nurses' notes, and any other notes that may appear on the computer. Then decisions are then made as to the patient's care for the day, or possible discharge. Most patients are referred to a subspecialist after being admitted, and a lot of the care is directed by his or her department. The hospitalist in charge of a patient, or the fourth-year resident, acting as attending, has the final word, however. This system works pretty well, but there is less direct contact with the patient's family and much greater reliance on the subspecialists, the laboratory studies, imaging, and technical studies. Also, there is little, if any, contact with anyone who knows the family, such as the generalist pediatrician who supplies the outside care of the patient. There is also less training for the residents on taking a good history, doing the physical exam, and the direct observation of the patient, and much less talking to the parents of the patient. There is more emphasis on the function of the various body systems than on the patient as an individual.

Because I made rounds for over fifty years at Oakland Children's Hospital, I tried to reverse or at least point out the problems with this gradual change. When I came, as the attending for the month to teach the residents, I insisted on seeing all the patients while making rounds, and on many occasions, we found things that had been overlooked and situations that demanded a different approach to the care of the child. My resident teams were impressed with what I could do without as much of the technical support on which they relied so heavily. They, however, had little

confidence in their own ability to develop the skills they would need in a private practice in the community, where the practitioner requires much less technical support.

A number of cases in which I have been involved are pertinent to my comments. The pediatric hospital in Philadelphia was, at that time, located in the heart of a very low-income area. Most of our families were thus Afro-Americans. One day, while making rounds, one of the nurses came over and told me that a little four-year-old was very unusual. "He can read and do arithmetic, and he is calling attention to our intravenous lines when they are running out." It turned out that his family knew all about it. The mother said, "Yes, he knows a lot about everybody and everything, and he won't keep his mouth shut. He's going to become king of the rackets." He turned out to have a very high IQ. One of our residents told us that he belonged to a group that followed kids like this and tried to be sure that they didn't get into gangs and got a good education. Many years later, at Oakland Children's Hospital, a little patient, with a viral respiratory infection, and again about four years old, greeted me on rounds by saying, "How am I? What's my temperature, and can I go home?"

I asked how he felt, and he replied that he felt fine. I turned to talk to his mother and he said, "She doesn't speak English. You tell me and I will tell her."

Again he turned out to be a very smart child who was going to require guidance and a good education. Dr. Feynman, the American physicist, was so brilliant in high school that his teachers were afraid that his family might not send him to college, since no one in his family had done so. They pleaded with his parents that he must go and offered help to be sure he did.

Another kind of problem was a child who had been resuscitated from a drowning accident about six months before. Unfortunately, although his various organs were working well, his brain was not. His father and an aunt who were taking care of him felt very guilty and wanted everything done that could be done. For six months he had been in a teaching hospital, and the various specialists had seen to it that all had been well taken care of, although his brain was not working. His family had received no psychiatric help, and were not aware that there was little or no hope of recovery. There really was no one to represent the family, and also to be involved in his care. We arranged for psychiatric help for the family and had him transferred to a facility more suited to his care. A generalist involved with the family would, I think, have changed his care at an earlier stage, and would have been of more help to the family than we were.

Another situation, in which I was involved, might have been prevented if I had been more alert. One of my patients was badly burned in a fire. She survived and required prolonged and extensive hospital care with multiple skin grafts. She had been a lovely young girl, and the parents were a very handsome couple. As time went by, it became obvious that she would survive but with a lot of scarring, and would always require a great deal of care. The family decided that they no longer needed my help and asked me to discontinue visiting her in the hospital. Within a week, after I was no longer her attending, she died. The only finding on post-mortem exam was an inexplicably high blood level of potassium. Although this may have been a hospital error in compounding her IV fluids, I felt that I should have pushed the parents to get psychiatric help in handling their feelings about her serious injury, and thus I might have been of more help to everybody.

Deliberate injury to children is not as uncommon as one might think, and the use of room cameras in hospitals has revealed more than we had expected. Primary care doctors are more likely to be aware of social and family problems and referral to Child Protective Services can often be a real help. The use of cameras opens up a lot of legal problems and is no longer done, or so I am told.

Another child was admitted when I was the attending physician, and we were making rounds. An IV was placed while the mother was at the bedside, and the nurse left the room to attend to some other duty. We later found out that the child was said to be quite retarded and was admitted for evaluation studies. In the half hour before we examined the boy, his heart suddenly ceased beating and attempts to revive him failed. Again, the autopsy failed to show a cause of death except for a very high level of potassium. This child had been admitted several times before, but though we had suspicions, nothing definite was found to indicate anything except an unfortunate accident with the compounding of the IV fluids.

A third child's story might have ended differently if a family pediatrician had been involved in her care. A young female child was admitted to my service with a history of episodes of unconsciousness, brief and without seizures. She seemed to be in good health, and nothing helpful was revealed on physical exam or laboratory work except that a request for consultation by the gastrointestinal service led to a test that seemed to indicate gastro esophageal reflux. Although this convinced them that this was the cause of her problems, I was not convinced. While the child was in the hospital, she had an episode accompanied by strange noises noted by the mother of another patient in the same room. This mother called the nurse, and though the patient's mother was at her bedside, she had not do so. I became suspicious that this might be a situation of maternal abuse and requested a psychiatric consult. No evidence was produced, but it was suggested that the family be referred to

Child Protective Services. Meanwhile, my gastrointestinal consultants remained convinced that this was gastro esophageal reflux and wished to do surgery to correct this. I thought the evidence for this was skimpy, and based on only one test. The family did not have a primary physician. I wished to have the child followed in our outpatient clinic and also referred her to Child Protective Services. About two weeks later, I got a call from a physician in another hospital's emergency room. She had had another episode of difficulty, but they could find nothing on exam or on laboratory work. I suggested that Child Protective Services should be informed. That did not happen, and instead she was admitted to our hospital on the gastroenterology service and the surgery was done. Three to four months later, the psychiatrist at Children's Hospital, whom I had consulted, called to tell me that the child had been sent to the hospital but was dead on arrival. I was never told what the autopsy revealed, if anything. I have used these cases as a prelude to a dissertation on what I feel is wrong, in my opinion, with the direction in which our medical care has been moving. As you can see, from the outline of my medical career, I have had the opportunity to observe and participate in the medical world for about seventy-three years. I practiced full time as a general pediatric practitioner in a small group for thirty-five years in Berkeley, CA, and spent a month each year for fifty-four years as a teacher of pediatric residents at Oakland Children's Hospital. I also participated for a few years in academia and remain an associate clinical professor of pediatrics at the University of California in San Francisco. In addition to teaching, after retirement from full-time practice, I have worked as a "locum tenens" for a small pediatric group in the mountains of northern California. (A "locum tenens" means a substitute for a physician who is not available.) I also worked for brief periods for the U.S. Public Health Service in a clinic in Kayenta on the Navajo reservation, and for a little less than a year, for Kaiser in Oakland, California.

Medical care has changed a great deal since I entered the profession seventy-three years ago. We have gradually changed from physicians who talked to parents about their children, diagnosed their illnesses, immunized them, and tried to keep them out of the hospital. We are now a profession dedicated to the treatment of diseases and the changes of disordered human physiology produced by congenital abnormalities, premature birth, disease, age, or trauma. Technology has revolutionized medical care and the treatment of disease. Research has continually shown us new ways to treat patients and the development of new drugs and treatments has increased the costs of medical care beyond belief. The primary care physicians were once treated with great respect for their ability to inform about illness and their efforts to care about and for their patients. They are now more valued as purveyors of medications and a conduit to specialists. The payments, especially for preventive care, are not great, and preventive medical care is often not covered by for-profit insurance companies. Psychological help often never reaches those who suffer, not from disease, but from the "slings and arrows of outrageous fortune," and the vicissitudes of our modern society, financial and medical. I recently noted the sad increase in the suicide rate of the middle-aged. It would seem that the burden of life is more than can be handled by an increasing number of us. Surely we can offer more!

The medications presented, on television and on the Internet are presented as miracles and all the possible side effects are covered at the end, very rapidly, and with no attempt to report on their likelihood or seriousness; only with the suggestion that you should "ask your doctor, if it's right for you." You might do better to talk to your pharmacist first.

My friends, who are in active practice as generalists for children or adults, complain about the use of the computer. It has many advantages, but it seems to reduce the time they spend with patients and the number they can see in a day. They also seem to spend a lot of time during a visit typing into the computer rather than talking with eye contact to the mother or patient. At least, with the computer, you can read their notes. We had a neurosurgeon who was unable to read his own notes, let alone anybody else's.

Primary care pediatricians are the lowest-paid physicians, and general practitioners are not much better off. Our specialists know more and more about less and less and it seems will eventually know everything about nothing, and our generalists, of course, will know nothing about everything. Seriously, the basic needs of human beings have not changed much, and they are not being met by our present system of care, which is not health care, it is illness care.

Complementary and alternative medicine have become increasingly a part of medical care in this century. The NCCIH (the National Center for Complementary and Integrative Health) reported that their study showed that 83 million people in this country, during the year 2007, had some contact with alternative care. About 40 billion was spent out of pocket for this as part of our 2.2 trillion dollars in total health care spending, about 1.5% of our total healthcare expenditures, and 11.2% of our out-of-pocket expenses for health care. We also spend about 15 billion dollars for non-vitamin, non-mineral health care medication and about 12 billion dollars for non-MD medical practitioners.

As in our educational system, we increasingly expect more than can be delivered. How many of us are aware that about a third of the money we spend on medical care is spent in the last few weeks of life? It doesn't make sense, but we have not done anything about it. Although hospice care is available most everywhere, it is not promoted and not used as much as it should be. Infants born with abnormalities incompatible with life are treated to the best of our ability regardless. I ran a perinatal mortality and morbidity committee for many years at a local hospital. Its purpose was to investigate the infant deaths that came shortly after birth in order to uncover the causes, and what, if anything, could we have done to prevent them. One fetus was known to have no brain, which was discovered in the last trimester of pregnancy when abortion can be difficult to obtain. Such babies will often live three or four months if fed and cared for. It was listed as stillborn, which is unusual, and so I asked how come? The obstetrician said, "The fact that I had a hand firmly over the newborn's mouth and nose may have had something to do with it." That would probably not happen today. In a medical climate where a large group of people would like to legally have life begin at conception, such children are delivered and kept alive for as long as they can breathe, which is often many months. Third-trimester abortions are presented as "terrible" with no redeeming qualifications. I served on a few committees and many who held fundamentalist religious beliefs frequently made it impossible to lay out programs that provided help for those in the greatest need. There was often no road to compromise. A House of Representatives member once said, "Right-to-lifers believe that life begins at conception and ends at birth," and there is some truth in that. I also remember a great example of hypocrisy when a purveyor of then illegal abortion was threatened with indictment. He said, "Okay, but if you indict me, I open my books." He was not indicted.

When I was chief resident at Philadelphia Children's Hospital, one of our residents asked our wonderful lady cardiologist a difficult question. "Why are we keeping this infant alive? The baby has only a three chambered heart and cannot survive. Why don't you stop our various life support systems and provide a peaceful end?"

She replied, "I agree with you completely. *You* do it." The care for the baby remained unchanged.

Our ethical problems constantly increase, and we generally don't want to think about them. The new gene editing technique, Crispr-Cas 9, presents abilities and potentials that need to be thoroughly evaluated and examined before "we are in over our heads." It is a discovery that has the potential to allow us to remove, with great precision, genes we don't like, and replace them with ones we do. This could be a great blessing in the elimination of many terrible illnesses. It also raises a multitude of ethical questions of its possible misuse.

The new outbreak of the Zika virus, spread by mosquitoes and seemingly causing all sorts of fetal brain defects, will raise many ethical questions concerning what we can do and what we should or should not do. In the last several years, young residents have asked me if I would enter the medical profession now, as I did seventy-three years ago. My answer is unequivocally yes. If you are oriented to research, this is a remarkable time to enter the field of genetics or any electronic field related to medicine. It would seem that the explosion of genetic information will be a two-edged sword. Genetic testing is becoming available at a price that already has come down to the point where it is increasingly offered, and not only to the wealthy. If insurance is to cover medical care inclusive of genetic care, the future presents a huge leap in medical costs and will require a great deal of supervision by either government or an outside committee.

If you like people, a clinical medical practice is very rewarding. We homo sapiens have not changed a bit, at least not yet. It is true that we are tribal, cantankerous, contumacious, combative, religious animals, and that our trust in myths and beliefs is greater than our trust in reason and science. However, our needs and concerns are basically the same as they have always been. It is also true you probably won't get rich, but you will still earn the love and respect of your families, your work will be varied and interesting, and you will do well enough financially to do very well in our present culture, whichever way it goes. Although I was never attracted to any of the subspecialties, I am sure they will continue to offer rewards to those they attract.

From my experience over an unusually long medical career, I have contemplated a number of problems with our current system of medical care. Our system of care is much too expensive and does not offer greater health or longevity than the systems in other countries. The countries that seem to handle health care better than we do are generally small and do not think of medical care as a "for-profit industry." Their populations are much more homogenous than ours, and their economies and politics more socialistic. We like to think of ourselves as a capitalist country, and to regard capitalism as superior to socialism in all regards. Of course, our public schools, police, fire departments, military, etc., are all socialistic as is much of our medical care for veterans, the elderly, the very poor, the Native Americans, the handicapped, and the incapacitated. In the treatment of serious illness, and the rapidity of obtaining care for serious complaints, we do quite well, that is if you have enough money. Although no one is left to die in the streets, it is a very inefficient and expensive way of providing even illness care, and it actively discourages preventive health care. Also I note that with the FEHBP (Federal Employee Health Benefit Plan)—although it is not a single-payer plan and is not free—all employees of the government and members of our House of Representatives and our Senate are covered by this plan and over 300 insurance companies compete for it. It is by far the best offer for the best price and available only to the government employees, and there is free help in choosing what is best for you.

My personal experience reveals the problems with care for many of us. I had a hernia repaired, which is not a challenging problem. I went to the outpatient surgical department of our local hospital at seven in the morning. I was not admitted to the hospital, although my surgeon, because of my age, would have been happier if I were admitted, just in case of trouble. I was admitted to outpatient surgery, a little after 7 a.m., and rested in bed for about an hour or so, with an IV in my arm and an interesting plastic disposable cover to keep me warm. The nurse checked my temperature, pulse, and blood pressure. At nine o'clock, I was taken to the operating room, lightly anesthetized, and operated upon. At about ten o'clock, I was back in the outpatient unit, and at eleven thirty, I was sent home. I later received a summary of my Medicare bill. The bill, which did not include the bills for the surgeon or the anesthesiologist, was for $35,000. Out of curiosity, I called Medicare and asked them about it. I was told that they, of course, would pay only about a quarter of that, but if I had no insurance, I would be responsible for the whole thing. This also would be a debt that I could not remove by bankruptcy. A hernia is a nuisance that is not life-threatening, unless intestinal obstruction occurs, and so, without insurance, or with a very high deductible or copay, I would likely put up with it and not get it repaired. A certain percentage of minor things like this do, if not repaired, lead to more severe problems, and if this happens, lead to the emergency room and the hospital. So, here we have a difference in medical care between the rich and the poor. Procrastination in care, not filling a prescribed medication, and not getting timely help tends to be attractive to many people. If your finances are limited and you are not within a reasonable distance for care, procrastination is also attractive. The laws of some states, which tend to remove clinics such as Planned Parenthood, add to the problems of poverty and increase the costs of Medicaid. Our local children's hospital provides care for a very varied population, which includes a lot of poor working-class families and some children who are not citizens and have no insurance. If a child is not insured and is not on Medicaid, the hospital may be able to have him placed there retroactively; if not, he is treated, and the hospital assumes the costs of care. If, over a period of time, the hospital faces bankruptcy, it may have to close. Fortunately, our children's hospital was taken over by the University of California Medical School in San Francisco and bankruptcy was avoided. It is the taxpayer who pays for all this in the long run, and thus we have a poor type of expensive "socialized" medical care for the poor and disadvantaged. We do provide care for all serious illness, but we treat the uninsured and the poor in a financially, unequal, and very inefficient system.

While I was working as a "locum tenens" (in place of) on the late shift, a father of an infant, who had been seen in the office the day before, called the office at 7:15 p.m. because he was worried that his baby might not be getting enough water, and was still having diarrhea. The nurse said, "We close at 8:00 p.m. Shall I send him to the ER?"

I said, "No, tell him to come in."

We had seen the baby the day before and had weighed him and found him to be active and vigorous and well hydrated. On this visit, we found that he had lost no weight and was thus not dehydrated; he looked vigorous and alert and his urination was also normal in frequency. We reassured the father, gave him more instructions about giving liquids, and made an appointment for the next day. Total cost for our visit was fifty-eight dollars. I talked to a colleague, who worked in the emergency room, and we calculated what the cost would be if he had gone there. The first problem was that the ER would have no knowledge of the baby, his illness, or his previous weight. After the usual history and exam, they would need to start an IV, get a blood count, and perform blood chemistries to be sure the child was not dehydrated nor his blood too acidic from the diarrhea. If the results were all normal, he would go home but with a charge of $520.

We are opening an increasing number of urgency clinics, which are much less expensive to operate than emergency rooms, because they don't have to take care of serious and life-threatening situations, and can handle patients on a walk-in basis. The so-called working poor tend to use the emergency room as the family doctor, which is very expensive, as I have shown. We have also found out that we need a huge number of additional general practitioners, or well-supervised nurse practitioners, or probably both. I have had contact with nurse practitioners in urgency clinics, which are not supervised by physicians on the premises. Our usual answer to questions about care was "Hold him, or her, closer to the phone. I can't see him." They would then send the patient over for us to see. We need to pay general pediatric and adult practitioners a lot more. It is a great advantage to have a doctor who knows you and/or your children, and is available when you are in need of care, and it is much less expensive than emergency rooms, and he or she can also provide a lot of preventive health care directed to your individual needs.

The medical care on the Indian reservations is run by the US Public Health Service. The service has its own Uniformed American University of Health Care as well. Young men or women may wish to investigate this as a route to becoming a medical professional without acquiring a lot of debt. After internship and residency training, a physician can agree to serve on the Indian reservations. They are supplied with housing, are paid a reasonable salary, and twenty thousand dollars a year off their student debt is paid by the government.

Having spent five and a half years in the army, I would rather make a deal with the Public Health Service and have student loans paid off than go into the military services, but that is also an available route. My experience, serving at the Kayenta clinic on the Navajo reservation for brief periods after I retired from private practice, was interesting and rewarding, and my pediatric abilities were put to good use. For the first time I encountered graduates of osteopathic medical schools, and found them to have excellent clinical abilities as general practitioners. Their training was less technical and more related to general practice than specialties. The nearest public health hospital was 76 miles away, in Tuba City, but physicians in the various specialties were available by phone for advice. Most of the physicians at the Kayenta clinic were just out of their resident training, and were thus very competent in their treatment of illnesses in general. The neonatal infant death rate, on the reservation, was lower than the national average, I think because they were almost all delivered at the hospital in Tuba City and received good prenatal care.

We all took nighttime calls and once I was especially grateful for telephone help. A lady came in, nine months pregnant and having abdominal cramps. I had not delivered a baby since medical school, and I did not want to start now. In an emergency, we could send her to the religious group, which ran a clinic and delivered babies at the four corners 15 miles away. I called the hospital at Tuba City, more than 70 miles away, to talk to the obstetrician. She said, "Run a strip." I said, "What is that?"

I was told, "Tell the nurse. She knows what to do." I did; the nurse did know, and ran a strip. I was then told to hold it up and tell her what I saw. I did and she then said, "You have it upside down; turn it over." I did so and reported what I saw. She then told me that the woman was not in labor, but since she was about to be, I should send her up by ambulance to Tuba City anyway. Needless to say, I was much relieved.

The Navajo reservation is large, 27,000 square miles, about the size of Massachusetts, Connecticut, and Rhode Island all together. In the 1860s, about 9,500 Navajo were forced to walk 400 miles, led by Kit Carson, to Bosque

Redondo. The Diné, the name the Navajo use for their people rather than "Navajo," lost many on the "long walk," and they considered the area near Fort Sumner to be a prison and they hated it. The traditional Diné construct an octagonal dwelling on their land called a "hogan," which always faces east and is destroyed after they die. When a baby is born, they bury the umbilical cord near their hogan, and thus consider themselves permanently attached to the land. They also have four sacred mountains in their area: San Francisco, Hesperus, Bianca, and Taylor. So, as you can see, they are very attached to their desert land, even though they were originally Athabaskan Indians who came south from northern Canada. The civil war general, Philip Sheridan, was assigned to find a reservation for them and he did. He told the president that their reservation was perfect for the Diné, and no one else would want to live there, since it is mostly a brown desert, and thus the Diné were returned to what they regarded as home.

The Navajos lifestyle is very unlike that of the Pueblo, who number about 15,000 and whose reservation is inside the Navajo reservation. The Pueblo live in clusters of dwellings and so close together that they share walls. Some ancient *anasazi* or Pueblo dwellings were built on high cliffs accessible only by climbing using hand holds. It is said that this protected them from Navajo raiders. The Pueblo claim to have taught the Diné how to raise sheep and to have, thus, civilized them.

The Navajo like to live about 15 miles from their nearest neighbors, if possible. Medical care runs into some special problems peculiar to them. When allowed to occupy the reservation, their population thrived, and they now number, as of 2015, about 350,000. Many do not live on the reservation and have melted into our society, but about 250,000 do. Some Diné patients come from outside the reservation because, they say, the medical care is good and free.

Since the present population of the Diné is from such a small gene pool, the number of congenital abnormalities is increased by inbreeding, even though the Diné have very strict rules as to which Diné tribes can intermarry. A common example of this is small amounts of blood in the urine exam noted on lab tests in many of them. I was told by my colleagues not to worry about that; it was common and did not indicate kidney disease. Since most of the patients lived at quite a distances from the clinic, and since the reservation did not have telephone service except in government buildings, it was necessary to make decisions about treatment and to do any tests at the time of the visit. If diagnosis and treatment depended on delayed results such as bacterial cultures, a nurse had to be sent out to bring the patient back or deliver the treatment necessary. I assume, however, that the smartphone has changed all that. Since the Diné were a hunter gatherer Athabaskan tribe for thousands of years, and since the amount of time between meals was very irregular and often long, the present population tends to have developed a slightly high blood sugar to protect them if food is scarce. They are thus more likely, when exposed to the modern American diet, complete with high-sugar drinks, to develop type 2 diabetes.

I used to wonder if the use of carrying boards for the infants would slow down their development. The infants spent a lot of time strapped on to the boards and leaning against walls. They seemed happy and alert, and it did not seem to slow them down at all. I asked one mother of a child we treated for a strep throat why she came to the clinic and also had a sand painting health ceremony. Her belief was that we treated the symptoms and made the sore throat go away, but the Diné medicine man's ceremony was concerned with the basic cause of the disease and health of the child.

Sand painting is a religious ceremony. The paintings are in color in the sand, and when completed, the patient is placed in the center of the painting to absorb the force connecting him or her to the universe and health. At the end of the ceremony, the sand from the painting is buried near the hogan and thus back to the earth. The Diné did not seem to be against immunizations to prevent disease, however.

Alcohol is a big problem in many of the people. It is forbidden to be sold on the reservation, and so many of the Diné go to the border of the reservation, where liquor stores are abundant, and drive home. Kids often ride in the back of a pickup, and if there is an accident, the clinic is overwhelmed with injured kids. Fortunately that did not happen while I was there.

One young woman who came in for treatment of a minor complaint and some general advice told me, when I advised her against Navajo fry bread, "I work in Flagstaff and eat a general American diet. I don't eat any of that stuff." She represented the one hundred thousand Navaho who live outside the reservation. As you can see, the various Native Americans represent special medical problems not easily taken care of by one system of care. The native people in Alaska and Hawaii and in the territories held by us also present special problems in medical care offered by the public health service. Many religious groups in the United States also see medical care differently, such as the Hutterites, Amish (now about 300,000 in the United States), the Bruderhoff, and other Mennonites. The "Seventh-Day Adventists," for example, will not accept treatment with human products such as blood transfusions and gamma globulin. Since we do not deny care to any who appear at our various clinics, offices, and emergency rooms, we need to have a system that is inclusive, and we need to give more thought to how best to provide care at a reasonable expense for all of us.

I had one patient who had Kawasaki disease (a very severe inflammatory disease with serious heart problems), and the family were Seventh-Day Adventists. I talked with them about the immediate necessity for gamma globulin. I emphasized the risks of not giving it right now, and explained that so much was done to it that it was not the human plasma it started out as. This gave them the opportunity to decide that it was not a human product, and we were allowed to give it.

I also worked for Kaiser for several months after I had retired from my private pediatric practice. Kaiser represented a type of medical care on a large scale, which we had begun on a small scale. I had long ago realized that we, in the United States, were increasingly moving toward expensive "cover your ass" illness care. We physicians in California had urged and helped pass a bill, which restricted malpractice suits to $250,000 for non-economic damages such as pain and suffering. This was a big help and greatly reduced the number of malpractice suits. Despite this, many obstetricians gave up delivering babies and devoted themselves to gynecology. Their insurance premiums were colossal if they covered obstetrics. If a baby is not normal at birth, the obstetrician is often blamed regardless of the cause of the abnormality. Many physicians of all specialties have begun to perform studies, which are not really indicated, to protect themselves in case of a malpractice suit. My observation through the years has been that human beings, being what they are, act in predictable ways. The practice of medicine on a "pay per visit" basis, which is essentially a "for-profit business," has problems. It is more profitable to do more in the way of tests and studies and the use of equipment, such as electrocardiogram machines or others, which one may have in the office or clinic, than to not use them.

In teaching hospitals, the residents in training programs generally have no idea of the cost of the various tests that they order on their patients. For example, MRI imaging is very expensive, as are echo cardiogram tests, and many others, which are commonly ordered. The constant development of new tests and new machines and all our technological advances are wonderful, if properly used when necessary. The urge, however, is to overuse them. The patients, in general, have little control over what things are done for their benefit, or without much benefit, and usually information is not available as to which. Avarice and greed are not going to go away, and close regulation, even with the best intentions may not work well enough. The television advertisements and the alternative medical suggestions on the Internet are also a case in point. So-called alternative medicine has advanced by leaps and bounds and is not covered by any effective regulations or regulatory groups. The Internet provides remarkable information, which is very difficult to evaluate medically or otherwise. Much of the information is based on fear (serious illnesses for which conventional medicine has no effective treatment), distrust (the pharmaceutical industries don't want you to know), and biographical stories of miraculous cures, or cosmetic treatments to halt the deteriorating effects of age. Many pharmaceutical companies put on additional pressure by suggesting that you should ask your doctor "if this would be right for you." The fact that dietary supplements are not checked by any agency as to their potency or safety or effectiveness puts a great load on the consumer. It is discouraging to read that they often do not contain the amount they say they do, or worse, not the substance they say they do. The epitome of all this, is, "Let the buyer beware." It has always been so, but never with such a deluge of information and quackery.

The rise in the number of anti-immunization groups has led many of my colleagues to refuse to accept families who won't be immunized. Some school districts also have excluded children from school, unless immunized. Measles, which had become a rare problem, has come back with occasional outbreaks among mostly non-immunized patients and leads to serious complications such as inflammation of the brain (encephalitis). Many of the people who are against immunizations are convinced that the measles vaccine is responsible for autism, even though this has been extensively studied and shown to be not so. Rubella (German measles) is only a significant problem if you happen to be pregnant. It causes congenital abnormalities in the fetus, as does the newly prominent Vinka virus. Many families who sit in a waiting room worry about exposing their children to others who may have a contagious disease. Whooping cough has returned in a few young infants, and some older children and adults. It is not as severe in the adult population but gives a prolonged cough that is often not diagnosed correctly. The last immunization used to be at age five and is now given in the teens. The newer pertussis (whooping cough) vaccines give many fewer reactions but are not as potent and don't last as long. Also, antibodies used to be present in mothers who had had various childhood diseases. This is often no longer true, and so the newborn baby, in the developed countries, no longer receives them by way of the placenta, nor in the breastmilk. Thus, young infants have no protection for the first four months until they complete some of their immunizations, such as DPT. Because of this, adults are now urged to get a whooping cough booster combined with their diphtheria and tetanus booster. It needs to be repeated every ten years or so to maintain the immunity. A grandparent with a prolonged cough may visit a new infant in the family, not yet immunized, and usually they do not realize what they have. Most of our adult physicians (internal medical specialists and general practitioners) have never seen whooping cough. This has led to a return of a disease very nasty and dangerous to small infants as it can produce brain damage or be fatal. England, for a period of a few years, discontinued the use of pertussis vaccine. The disease had become a rarity and the vaccine caused many reactions, so it seemed reasonable. Unfortunately, the whooping cough came rapidly back and caused many deaths and severe brain damage among some small infants, and so it was quickly restarted. The vaccine has been improved, and so it causes fewer reactions than the old vaccine, but it does not provide a long lasting protection. Pediatricians, thus, are concerned about the safety of their waiting rooms, and who is sitting in them.

Our access to information turns out to be a two -edged sword. It dates back to a time of great fear of contagious disease. Children were once quarantined for many of the diseases we now immunize against, and many families would not let their children swim in public pools because of polio. How quickly we forget!

Although we now have a multitude of antibacterial medications, the bacteria, which reproduce about every eight hours, has evolved strains resistant to our antibacterial drugs and combinations thereof. Staphylococcal bacteria and tuberculosis bacteria are examples. The unnecessary use of antibacterial drugs in cattle and other animals has made this a lot worse. Hospitals also have become a place where one is likely to be infected with bacteria that are hard to treat.

This year a bacteria was found resistant to all antibiotics and combinations of them. They reproduce and evolve faster than we can produce antibacterial drugs. We are getting back to where we were eighty years ago when our defense against only a few contagious diseases, e.g., smallpox and rabies, was immunization. I also have to point out to many families that the *T* in DPT immunization stands for tetanus, which is not a contagious disease, and so there is no herd immunity in the general population.

Most advanced countries have developed so-called single-payer medical care systems and many developing countries have done likewise. In the United States, these systems are called "socialized medicine," and this is considered a derogatory appellation. We, in fact, have created a triple system. Single payer or socialized medicine is provided by, Medicare for the elderly, Medicaid for the poor, and public health medical care for the Native Americans. We also provide government medical service, or socialized medical care, for veterans and special help for those who are disabled or handicapped and require help to survive and overcome their disabilities. These are all examples of socialized medicine. Such programs are well appreciated, but they are very expensive primarily because they make use of a capitalist for-profit system to provide care and they do not allow the programs to bargain with the pharmaceutical companies for prices of drugs. That is, in part, why drugs are much cheaper in Canada and Mexico. Also, the extension of patents on drugs prolongs the arrival of generic drugs in our drugstores.

Many years ago a few people tried to promote a different kind of care. Health maintenance organizations were started in this country in the 1920s and are of many different types. Some HMOs are so-called closed-panel systems. In these, the physicians are hired by the organization, and usually, to see a specialist, you must be referred by your primary care doctor. There are about 450 HMOs in the USA. PPOs allow you to go directly to a specialist, rather than be referred by your primary physician. The Kaiser Permanente plan is a closed-panel plan, and thus you must be referred by your primary physician if you need to see a specialist. Also you are restricted to physicians in the system. Henry Kaiser started a business career, which had involved him in dam building and other construction products. His great success came in World War II and involved welding ships rather than using rivets. He established a number of shipyards using this technique, and his greatest one, in Richmond, California, set a record of 4 days and 15 hours from laying the keel to launching the ship. He was very concerned with

helping the refugees trying to escape from the terrors of World War II, and also constructing ships to carry war materials to Europe and troops to Asia. His shipyards not only turned out merchant vessels very rapidly using relatively unskilled labor, they also turned out small aircraft carriers. Mr. Kaiser decided to create Kaiser Permanente to provide medical care for his employees. This was not regarded favorably by the local medical community, and was thought to be inferior medical care, but it soon spread to involve patients from the surrounding communities and was gradually accepted as a permanent part of the medical communities in California.

The idea of prepaid medical care with its own hospitals and physicians on salary, or HMOs, started in the 1920s, almost 100 years ago. In recent years they have become increasingly popular. They vary in many ways, and it is important to study them and find what suits you. They all have deductibles and copays and other slight differences. They are a compromise between a for-profit system and a socialized single-payer government system.

Kaiser is mostly in California, and although each independent clinic is physician owned and operates as a for-profit, its dominant payer is the Kaiser Health Organization, which is nonprofit. It numbers 10 million members, 39 hospitals, with a new 400-bed one in San Diego, California, and there are 618 clinics, 17,000 physicians, 48,000 nurses, and 174,000 employees. Of the top urban health centers in the USA, one-third are Kaiser-owned. My experience at Kaiser raised a number of questions, but they seemed to be well organized and run the system quite well. They were well aware that preventive medical care, if properly used, could reduce costs, and they provided all physicians, including their residents in training, with a list of costs of all laboratory tests, visual screenings, and medical machine tests. They also use physicians' assistants and nurse practitioners to provide a lot of preventive care, and I am told that they also have bargaining power with drug companies for lower drug costs because of their size and volume of business. (as I said, Medicare is forbidden to bargain with drug companies).

Their physicians compare well, in training and experience, with the practitioners in the general community. However, to get good care, you need to have a primary physician, and know how the system works. I found that a large number of patients had no primary physician. Many used to have, but he or she either retired or died or left Kaiser. I told them all that they needed to have and ask for their primary physician, and to avoid the urgency clinics unless it was truly urgent and their primary doctor was not available. The response I usually got was a request: "Can you be our primary pediatrician?" I, of course, could not be as I was not a full-time Kaiser doctor. I also noted that their doctors in the urgency clinics were mostly young, and many were moonlighting as a temporary additional job but also had other positions. My feeling was that they needed better supervision in the urgency clinics from more experienced physicians. If you had a primary physician and worked the system properly, however, Kaiser provided good care and much more preventive health care than most medical groups or individual practitioners.

Basically all medical care comes down to the primary care physicians, and their competence and dedication. If what is offered does not suit the patient and the physicians, it won't survive.

There has been a huge change in those giving the care. Our society has changed, and women physicians, in general, have a very different outlook than male physicians. They are much more interested in their ability to control their work hours and able to thus arrange their lives to the necessity of multitasking. Raising a family and the obligations of maintaining a home have always been more a female than male concern. I have seen an increasing number of families where the male, or partner, has taken over the primary home making, child raising, and housework activities, but this is not the usual. This has led to physicians moving to more easily regulated positions, as emergency room physicians, hospitalists, specialists or working for HMOs.

As a pediatrician, I spent my life dealing primarily with women, and in many ways my work was closer to that of a veterinarian than the doctors who cared for adults. Also, I spent the majority of my time treating minor illnesses and advising parents about developmental problems and the prevention of illness. Our patients were mostly from a very academic community and a large number were connected to the university. After all, we were referred to as "The People's Republic of Berkeley." Our work was

primarily preventive and we rarely had to hospitalize a child. Our practice grew well and we were well accepted by the community. Capitation (the word used by HMOs to describe prepay medical care) is still quite popular in California and Oregon, but not in the rest of the country. It is most popular in areas where HMOs are popular. Capitation in California was 29 percent in 2008 and in Oregon, 18 percent. The rest of the country about 4 percent. It was much more popular in the 1990s and its popularity has dropped since then. It proved to be discouraging to both patients and caregivers. Physicians were making less money than with pay-per-visit medical care, and patients felt that the care provided was perhaps not as good, since although accepted by the medical societies, there is still a feeling that they do not provide as good medical care as the fee for service care. It was also not reducing medical costs as much as had been hoped. However, it is again on the increase, in part because of the continued rise in medical costs, and the increased government subsidies required to sustain the competition of private health insurance with Medicare and the other socialistic types of care. The providers and the patients have changed greatly in recent years. The majority of new physicians are women with a different attitude toward providing care, and our technology, both in treatment and prevention of disease, has developed tremendously and with great rapidity. Alternative medical care practitioners, with the help of the Internet and television, account for large out-of-pocket expenses. Nonvitamin and nonmineral products cost us about $15 billion a year, and an additional $12 billion is spent for non-MD practitioners, very little of which is covered by insurance.

My conclusion from all this experience is that for-profit medical care does not, and will not, work. It has led to illness care in preference to health care, and to the proliferation of unnecessary and misdirected care. Since 1970 the cost of private insurance has risen one percent per year, faster than Medicare. Over the next decade it is estimated that private care cost will grow 4.8 percent per year, Medicare 2.5 percent. Actually it is even worse than this. In the 1970s, insurance companies convinced the government that private Medicare could outcompete the government, and so it was allowed to try. A -5 percent of the Medicare payment was placed on their charges to see if the claim that they would be cheaper than standard Medicare was true. The insurance companies could not make a profit and gave up. The Medicare advantage plans came again in the 1990s, but without the 5 percent reduction and have, instead, been subsidized by the government so that by 2014, they were costing the government and subscribers combined 14.8 percent more than standard Medicare. The Affordable Care Act has gradually reduced the subsidies, and it is supposed to produce a level playing field by 2017. The political manipulation, including subsidies, with all of this, makes it very difficult for the average person to know who pays for what. Avarice and greed, however, do not go away.

We face an economy where more and more jobs are in the service industries and not in manufacturing. Robots in manufacturing are the future, and our loss of those jobs will continue regardless of how cheap labor is overseas. My belief is that the people who own the robots will make the money. The middle class will need to own a piece of the companies who own the robots or we will have big troubles. We need a move toward a single-payor government medical system with close supervision by competent people and laws that assure that health care is a right, not a privilege for those who can afford it.

The millennial generation is finding that good jobs and reasonable salaries require more than just a college degree. Medicine falls into that category. Our doctors should not strive to make a fortune in medical care, but rather to earn a salary commensurate with their abilities, education, and knowledge and to provide care and improved health for all.

SUGGESTIONS TO CONSIDER

Assuming that single- payer medical care is not going to happen overnight

1) Financial help - For physicians who are willing to organize clinics to replace emergency rooms for non-emergency visits of patients who are using emergency rooms as their family doctor.

2) Patients should have to pay a copayment if they use the emergency room rather than an urgency clinic or personal physician for routine non-emergency care.

3) The requirement that all citizens be covered by medical insurance of some kind should be continued, with provisions for illegal immigrants and the uninsured, which does not bankrupt hospitals. The experiences of the clinics and hospitals, such as Kaiser Permanente, Mayo, Cleveland, and many others, can be used for study as to what should and should not be done.

4) Increased compensation for general practitioners, general internists, and general pediatricians. Without this, or a flood of nurse practitioners, we do not have a sufficient force of physicians to do the job. If nurse practitioners are to be used in large numbers, they must be supervised by physicians, *on site and available for consultation, as with residents in training.*

5) Community practitioners should be brought back into the teaching hospitals as attending physicians. To do this, they should be paid a reasonable amount to cover the lost time from their offices. Fourth-year residents, who are now used as attending physicians, should be required to spend a month in a medical office, or outside clinic, as part of their training.

Hospitalists, who practice only in the hospital, should have scheduled time, with the community physicians, to discuss mutual problems relating to their patients. When a patient is admitted to the hospital, contact by phone with the referring physician should be made and any relevant information about the patient and the family should be a part of the hospital record.

6) Since it seems that single-payer medical care cannot be achieved in the USA at the present time, especially considering our present government, a cure for the present chaos of very expensive for-profit illness care combined with HMOs and government care will be difficult. The drop in the Canadian dollar and the reduced cost of medical procedures in Mexico, Europe, and Asia have prompted an increasing number of people to seek care, especially elective surgery, and prescription drugs, outside the USA. Obama care has proved to be a start in the right direction, but it needs to be reformed and not discarded. A general government care program should be offered in competition to the private medical insurance and on a level playing field, e.g., no subsidies, because the non-medical expenses of pharmaceutical companies, and insurance companies, such as advertising, have become outrageous and there is a constant urge to increase the profits. At the present

time, the insurance companies are offering more coverage of different procedures rather than lowering fees. Payment for drugs, dental care, oculists, etc. Different insurance companies try different coverages and scales to compete, and this leads to all sorts of aberrations in medical care. Government subsidies to "for-profit insurance companies" are an unnecessary expense especially to allow them to compete with Medicare, and do not offer a level playing field.

Expansion of prepaid medical care would reduce the urge to make use of facilities and equipment just because they are available, and produce income. Medicare and Medicaid should have the ability to negotiate with pharmaceutical companies as they do in single-payer countries such as Canada and Europe, and we need control of what is allowed to be advertised and how it is advertised on television and other electronic media. The Affordable Care Act is a step in the right direction, but if we would concentrate on preventive health care, illness care would be less of a problem and much less expensive. If our care in the USA encouraged people to use preventive health care and seek early help for problems and illnesses, we would save a lot of money.

7) Alternative medicine needs to be better evaluated, perhaps trying to decide who is licensed and who is not to provide health care. Medications that are sold as food supplements need to be controlled, as prescription drugs are, for possible harm and truth in packaging and content.

8) The availability of hospice care should be advertised much more than it is, and if the government were to subsidize prepay, nonprofit health care groups, rather than insurance companies, we could do a lot better for the health and happiness of our citizens. We need to bring the needs of people back into our health care and use some common sense about how we spend our money.

(9) In a general philosophical and social way, there needs to be much more discussion in our society and country about medical care. The technological and genetic advances are

moving so rapidly that much of what we are doing should be examined with great care by all of us. The care of the very severely compromised at birth and the very premature infants, coupled with the care of the dying elderly, consume a very large percentage of our medical expenses and are often not desired by the families or the patients, particularly in the care of the dying elderly. Our intensive care units are not appropriate care for many, especially the very elderly like me, but there is often no discussion prior to being placed there.

What I have written above shows a lot of things we could consider that would greatly reduce the cost of medical care in this country, but the main cause of expensive healthcare in the our country is that we prefer not to discuss it, and we generally consider illness care to be medical care. "If it ain't broke, don't fix it." We are a very diverse society, and we don't agree on many things. Religious beliefs are very varied, and many strongly religious groups believe that some things are just plain wrong and should not be allowed to be done by anyone.

When I was a young adult seventy years ago, there was little we could do to alter the various illnesses, and religious beliefs were not much of a factor in our medical care. I thus began my medical career just about at the start of the scientific medical revolution. Our attitude then toward science in general was very positive and quite accepting of any progress in medical care. It also began to be obvious that many so-called advances were not helpful. My young residents were increasingly curious about what we did when I was a resident in training and were horrified at many of the procedures, which we carried out to make a diagnosis and or to treat a sick patient. My reply was that I could understand their horror, but also I appreciated the likelihood that about 50 percent of what we do today is wrong, but we just don't know which 50 percent it is. At that time, we generalists also carried out procedures that would only be done by specialists today.

Our treatment of very small premature babies had changed in that we had incubators for the babies and oxygen to help with their difficulties in breathing. A very experienced nurse in the hospital nursery for very small premature babies used to pick them up and carry them around and croon to them. We asked our attending physician why this was allowed. His reply was interesting. He said that they had noted that babies in her care did better and were more likely to survive than those that were not. He said that when we asked her why that was so, her reply was, "I keep the resident's hands off the babies and provide time out of the damn machines for cuddling and human contact."

When I first joined the group, in practice mothers were not allowed to have the babies with them in their room. A new colleague in the group, about seven years after I joined the group, was upset by this, and he and I got the main delivery hospital, in Berkeley, to change its rules and allow what was called "rooming in A new colleague joined our group, about fifteen years after I had joined, and he had had training in a new specialty called neonatology. Thus began a new era of care for the newborn, especially the very small premature infants. We took care of full-term, or only slightly premature babies, and the neonatologists took care of the sick and the very premature. The arrival of this specialty signaled a new era in many ways. The care of small newborns improved greatly, and the expense of their care increased greatly; many very small babies survived who would not have survived in the past. We began to refer to them as "million-dollar babies." By that time, I had begun to chair the "Neonatal Mortality and Morbidity Committee." A few things became obvious. The babies who survived were getting smaller and smaller, the costs of their care were getting greater and greater, and only about one in four of those that survived developed without major problems. Therefore the expense of their lifetime care has added greatly to the costs of medical care.

The problems of medical ethics have also increased. With the advent of the Internet and the smartphone and our ability to express ourselves on Facebook or Twitter or to learn from Google or Wikipedia, we live in a new world.

Many beliefs, true or false, are strongly held. For example, if we were to accept that life begins at conception, abortion would be murder. Certain types of birth control would also be considered such. Many people no longer accept scientific evidence and make decisions based more on belief rather than scientific evidence or reasonable compromise. This does not lead to strong rational decisions for care. Immunizations are an example. To provide care for families opposed to immunizations is an increasing problem. Families who do not immunize find that their children often are not allowed to attend school. Immunizations have become many in number and expensive, and families with a tight budget may postpone them or refuse them. In short, decisions that we made decades ago are no longer considered valid. New discoveries are made daily, and our ability to debate their pros and cons cannot keep up. The pharmaceutical industry not only works hard at making new drugs, but the price of some treatments and medications are astronomical.

All the things I have mentioned lead us to the necessity, as a country with a democratic form of government, to thoroughly examine and think about our system of medical care. We no longer can afford to ignore what is happening in medical care, nor the growing disparity of quality care between the rich and the poor among our people. Our capitalistic economy is not sacrosanct, nor is our mixed private and government medical system.

Our medical system is a combination of many practitioners, regular MDs, (surgical and medical), doctors of osteopathy, skilled nurse practitioners, physical therapists, and others. In addition, we have alternative practitioners of many different kinds—homeopaths, naturopaths, chiropractors, midwives, and many others difficult to label. All these practitioners practice alone, in groups, or as salaried practitioners employed by groups. The training, the licensing, and the supervision of alternative medical people varies greatly and is often unknown to their clients. In addition, there are many different ways of paying practitioners. "For-profits" usually pay per visit; "nonprofits" usually prepay monthly or by the year. We have a variety of hospitals and groups of licensed physicians of various types, and we have government restrictions and laws that regulate the licensed. The licensing of alternative practitioners varies from state to state, and so does certification of various types of medical care. Regulation varies greatly among the states, and may not exist for some practitioners. Some are regulated by the state and some by private representatives of the various systems of care. Religious groups, such as Mary Baker Eddy's Christian Science Church, are not considered providers of medical care, nor are the Navajo sand painters. For-profit insurance companies pay for our medical care but with restrictions as to doctors, specialists, nurse practitioners, physical therapists, psychologists, chiropractors, and others, depending on the particular insurance policies, as do restrictions on care, copays, and deductibles. The government pays for care with Medicare for the elderly, Medicaid for the poor, Social Security for the disabled (along with disability insurance), veterans' medical care, and medical care for Native Americans and some residents of American possessions. As you can see, this conglomeration of care in the United States is very difficult to sort out or to control or regulate. It is almost impossible to evaluate economically, or for its effectiveness.

As I have pointed out, our drug industry is in a similar situation. As private companies, they have more or less complete control over the retail price of their products. Patented medications are protected for as long as the patents run and companies can charge whatever the traffic will bear. Lobbyists are constantly asking Congress to extend the period of time the patents run. This prevents competition from other companies to produce much cheaper generic drugs that are the same as the patented product.

Most supplements used by the alternative practitioners are regarded as foods and are not regulated by the FDA.

All this confusion about medical care points to a simple basic fact. We, as a country, have not made up our minds about medical care. Is it a basic right of people in a "civilized" society to receive medical care, or is it a privilege? If it is a basic right, how do we define medical care, how do we pay for it, and what is included or excluded? If we don't want government regulation of who gives care or who receives it, who else will supervise it and how? If we decide on "single-payer" government care, will we allow restriction of certain very costly methods of care at the discretion of patients, or their agents acting for them? For example, we now frequently use the intensive care unit for terminally ill patients, rather than a special unit in an institution, or home, designed to provide hospice care. At present, we do not advertise or really promote hospice care at home. Can we decide about the kind of care we provide our very small or very congenitally deformed babies who have no chance of living a normal life, but who are now treated with the use of every advanced technique available? I realize that these are very difficult questions to answer, and the use of ethics committees, although essential in dealing with these problems, will be called all sorts of names such as "death squads," murderers, atheists with no religious beliefs and no morals, etc. Still, if we want to maintain our research and progress in biological science, and solutions to our current problems both medical, financial, and ethical, it must be done.

As you can see, I am particularly worried about the loss of the personal touch and relationships in medical care. As we become increasingly involved in the treatment of illness, we have neglected, to some extent, the human or humane aspects of life. This shows up, not only in medical care, but in our social relationships as well. In contacts with people, I am troubled to find that folk from dictatorial or socialistic societies who have arrived in capitalistic countries such as ours say that they miss the strong social bonding of their former country. East Germans, when they came in contact with West German society, for example, and Cuban refugees in our country, as another example. Our society seemed to them cold, and an "every-one-for-him-or-herself society." I believe that this is especially important in medical care, and is lacking in our highly technical approach to medicine. This may be the reason for the expansion of alternative approaches to medical care in the USA, and the huge expansion of possible disease prevention by the use of herbal and dietary products.

www.ingramcontent.com/pod-product-compliance
Lightning Source LLC
Chambersburg PA
CBHW030854180526
45163CB00004B/1570